THE CONTEMPORARY A-Z ACNE REMEDY GUIDE

Discover Basic Effective Skin Care Tips for Combating Acne in Teens and Adults.

SANDRA DEBORAH

Thank you for your purchase.

I'd appreciate it if you could leave me some feedback, share your thoughts, and tell me about your Amazon experience.

HOW DO I WRITE A REVIEW?

- Sign in to your Amazon account

- Go to "Your Orders"

- Go to "This Product"

- Go to "Write a Product Review"

TABLE OF CONTENTS

INTRODUCTION

Acne is a skin disorder that affects the hair follicles as well as the oil glands. Pimples, black/white heads, reddishness, and cysts are all symptoms. Face acne can greatly impair on your appearance, while body acne can completely ruin your day by making you uncomfortable. Some people dismiss the topic of 'Acne skin care' because they consider acne to be a minor issue. The significance of 'Acne skin care', on the other hand, cannot be overstated.

CHAPTER ONE

WHAT IS ACNE AND HOW CAN I TREAT IT?

Acne skin care should begin well before the acne symptoms develop. It's more important to be proactive than reactive when it comes to acne skin care. Acne skin care is all about being aware of the precautions to take. Acne skin care entails strictly adhering to daily skin care practices. So, let's have a look at how we may incorporate "acne skin care" into our everyday regimen.

The most basic aspect of 'acne skin care' is hygiene. Showering in the morning is the most fundamental method of keeping the skin clean. Many people, in fact, take night showers (that not only help in keeping your skin clean but also provide relaxation to your body and enable a good sleep). If you live in a hot and/or humid climate, taking a night shower is a necessary. In fact, any exercise that results in excessive sweating should be followed by a shower. It's a highly successful method of 'acne skin care.'

Acne skin care, on the other hand, is more than just taking a shower. Wearing clean clothes and sleeping on clean pillows are other important aspects of acne skin care. Furthermore, overly tight clothing can cause sweat to collect fast; therefore, cotton clothing that is soft and comfy is preferable, especially if you have acne. In the same way, 'acne skin care' encourages you to clean your make-up brush and any other equipment you use on your body on a regular basis.

A moderate, water-soluble, oil-free, and soap-free cleanser should also be used to keep your face, neck, and arms clean. The most vital aspect of any acne skin care routine is cleansing. Cleaners are the simplest and most efficient way to remove debris, filth, pollutants, and excess oil from your skin, lowering your chances of developing acne. Acne skin care also recommended that you remove your make-up with a make-up remover before going to bed (not in the morning).

If you already have acne, avoid touching or squeezing it because this might result in permanent scarring. Using an over-the-counter drug and a clean/soft cotton pad, 'acne skin care' advises gentle scrubbing and cleaning of the affected region. Over-the-counter acne skin care creams and lotions are widely accessible (a lot of these acne skin care products are actually cleansers). Contact a dermatologist for 'acne skin care' advice and treatment if these 'acne skin care' techniques don't yield the desired outcomes.

CHAPTER TWO

EVERYTHING YOU NEED TO KNOW ABOUT FACIAL SKIN CARE

It's more a matter of discipline than anything else when it comes to 'facial skin care.' What you require is a facial skin care routine (and you need to follow the facial skin care routine with complete seriousness). So, let's have a look at what makes up a good facial skin care routine. To put it simply, a facial skin care routine may be broken down into four steps:

* Detoxification

* Toning

* Exfoliation

* Moisturizing.

The first step in every facial skin care routine is cleansing. Cleaning your skin helps to remove dust, pollutants, grease, and excess oil, preventing damage to your skin. Simply apply a decent washing lotion or cream to your face and neck and gently massage it into your skin with upward strokes. Wipe your face with a soft facial tissue or cotton wool in a gentle patting motion (do not rub). Cleaning should be done at least twice a day, in the morning (as part of a comprehensive facial skin care routine) and evening (as part of a complete facial skin care routine) (on a standalone basis). Cleansers that dissolve in water are the ideal to use in your facial skin care routine.

The next step in a facial skin care routine is to tone. However, this is a portion of the facial skin care routine that is optional. The majority of the time, good washing can compensate for toning. Toning aids in the removal of all traces of filth, grease, and cleaner. Instead of making toning a regular part of your facial skin care routine, you can do it on occasion, such as after being exposed to very harsh environmental/pollution conditions.

Exfoliation is, once again, a kind of optional step in daily facial skin care. Exfoliation, on the other hand, should be done at least once a week (or twice, depending on the skin type and the environmental conditions). Because the skin's natural tendency to replenish skin cells every 3 to 4 weeks, exfoliation has a place in the facial skin care routine. Exfoliation is a facial skin care method that aids the skin in its natural process by eliminating dead skin cells that clog pores. Excessive or harsh exfoliation, on the other hand, might harm your skin, so you must strike a balance.

Moisturizing is the next step in facial skin care. In fact, moisturizing is the most crucial aspect of any facial skin care regimen. Moisturizers help to keep your skin from drying out. Dry skin is undesirable because it causes the upper layer of skin to break down, resulting in the formation of dead skin cells. To make the moisturiser more effective, use mild upward strokes once more. Moisturizers are most effective when applied to warm, damp skin. So, in the preceding steps of your facial skin care routine, don't strive to eliminate all of the moisture.

Aside from your regular face skin care routine, you should also use the following facial skin care techniques:

* Rather than washing away your make-up, use a good make-up remover.

* When selecting facial skin care products, consider your skin type as well as the surroundings.

* Test a new facial skin care product on a small piece of skin, such as the ear lobes, before starting to use it.

* Don't scuff your skin too much.

* Use sunscreen products to protect yourself from the sun.

Everything you need to know about sensitive skin care

There are a few basic rules that govern 'sensitive skin care.' However, before we get into the sensitive skin care principles, it's crucial to understand what sensitive skin is. Sensitive skin is skin that cannot withstand any unfavourable conditions (environmental or otherwise) and is easily irritated by foreign elements (including skin care products). As a result, certain products are designated as sensitive skin care products. The degree of sensitivity, on the other hand, can differ from person to person (and depending on that, the sensitive skin care procedures vary too).

Detergents and other chemical-based products have a negative impact on all skin types. Damage, on the other hand, often begins after a set threshold is crossed (or tolerance level). For sensitive skin types, this tolerance level is quite low, resulting in skin that is easily and quickly damaged. Potential irritants are either avoided or kept at very low doses in sensitive skin care products.

Here are some delicate skin care suggestions:

* Only use sensitive skin products (i.e. the products that are marked for sensitive skin care only). Also, examine the product's instructions/notes to see if there are any specific restrictions/warnings).

* Even among sensitive skin care products, select the one with the fewest preservatives, colours, and other substances.

* Avoid using toners. The majority of them include alcohol and are not suitable for delicate skin.

* When conducting laundry or other chemical-based cleaning, wear protective gloves. If you have a rubber allergy, you can use cotton gloves underneath the rubber ones.

* Avoiding excessive sun exposure is another crucial recommendation for 'sensitive skin care.' Before going out in the sun, use sunscreen lotion.

* When caring for sensitive skin, it's also crucial to avoid exposure to dust and other contaminants. So, before you go out, make sure you're sufficiently covered.

* As a sensitive skin care product, use a hypoallergenic, noncomedogenic moisturizer (if there is none specifically labelled as a sensitive skin care product)

* Use non-soap, non-alcohol cleaners. When you get home from spending time outside, wash your face.

* Avoid exfoliating or scrubbing too forcefully. It might induce a tinge of redness as well as irritation.

* Do not wear your makeup for an extended period of time. Make use of makeup removers that are hypoallergenic.

As a result, sensitive skin care differs significantly from standard skin care. Sensitive skin care entails taking extra precautions with your skin (both in terms of sensitive skin care products and protection against environmental atrocities on skin).

CHAPTER THREE

SKIN CARE PRODUCTS THAT ARE ANTI-AGING

The song "forever young" comes to mind when I think of anti-aging skin care products. Anti-aging skin care treatments are extremely popular today; after all, who doesn't want to appear young for the rest of their lives?

When it comes to anti-aging skin care products, vitamin C-based anti-aging skin care products spring to mind first. These products function by allowing collagen to be synthesized (a structural protein that is found in skin). Anti-oxidants are linked to this category of anti-aging skin care products. Vitamin C-based anti-aging skin care solutions, on the other hand, run the risk of being oxidized themselves (as they come into contact with air during their usage). As a result, certain anti-aging skin care products are made from vitamin C compounds, which are more stable and less expensive. However, the efficacy of such anti-aging skin care products is not as high as that of vitamin C-based anti-aging skin care.

Vitamin E and lipoic acid, in addition to vitamin C, are anti-oxidants. Vitamin E is a fat-soluble antioxidant found in human blood that aids in the development of infection resistance. Vitamin E has also been linked to the prevention of cancer. Liponic acid is well-known for efficiently combating the effects of aging by correcting the skin damage produced by the aging process.

The other type of anti-aging skin care product is phytochemicals. Special substances collected from plants are known as phytochemicals. Phytochemicals are used in a wide range of applications nowadays. Prostate cancer, breast cancer, and colon cancer are among the cancers that phytochemicals help to prevent. As a result, they can be found in anti-aging skin care products.

Some B-vitamins, such as B5, B6, and B12, are also used in anti-aging skin care.

Anti-aging skin care products are a huge field that requires a great deal of research. Despite the fact that the currently available products are effective, they nonetheless face problems. Hopefully, these issues will be rectified in due time, allowing for better and less expensive anti-aging skin care solutions.

Anti-aging skin care products, on the other hand, should only be used as a supplement to natural skin and body care. Drinking plenty of water, getting a good night's sleep, exercising frequently, following a nutritious diet, and avoiding stress are all important ways to slow down the aging process. There is no anti-aging skin care product that can truly replace them.

CHAPTER FOUR

SKIN CARE FOR THE ELDERLY

Anti-aging skin care is one of the most fascinating topics in skin care. As we age, our skin's (and, indeed, our entire body's) natural defenses deteriorate. The term "anti-aging skin care" refers to the act of protecting your skin against the detrimental effects of aging. 'Anti aging skin care' aids in the preservation of a youthful and fresh appearance for a longer length of time. However, the term "anti-aging skin care" does not end here. 'Anti aging skin care' is about keeping your resistance to disease as well as maintaining your appearance (good looks). Despite the fact that anti-aging awareness has grown over time, many people are still unable to recognize the signs of aging (and hence are unable to determine if they are in need of additional anti aging skin care measures).

Baldness, forgetfulness, greying hair, wrinkle formation, loss of eyesight or hearing loss, and menopause are some of the apparent anti-aging signs that can help you plan and execute your anti-aging skin care approach. When one or more of these signs appear, it's time to raise the bar on anti-aging skin care. It's important to note that we're discussing the inclusion of new anti-aging skin care measures, not the start of 'anti-aging skin care' from scratch. 'Anti-aging skin care' begins long before the first signs of age appear. Building and maintaining a proper skin care practice much earlier in life is essential for serious anti-aging skin care (say in your teens). Anti-aging skin care does not imply the use of any unique skin care technique, but rather the diligent application of a standard procedure. The aging process can be slowed by eating a lot of fruits, avoiding stress, drinking enough of water, and employing natural medicines.

As soon as the first indications of age appear, you should begin utilizing anti-aging skin care products. Anti-aging skin care products abound on the market. In fact, there are so many anti-aging skin care treatments on the market that they will almost certainly find you before you do. Also, as people get older, their skin changes dramatically. As a result, you'll need to evaluate your existing skin-care routine to see if it's still effective, i.e., if it's still appropriate for your skin.

It's important to understand that aging is a natural process that has no way of being stopped. All of these anti-aging skin treatments can only aid to slow down the aging process.

CHAPTER FIVE

SKIN CARE THAT INHIBITS FAST AGING PROCESS

In today's environment, 'anti aging skin care' is a widely popular notion. Everyone nowadays seeks to conceal their age with anti aging skin care methods (and a number of people are successful too). However, there is no such thing as a miraculous medication for anti aging skin care. It's all about discipline when it comes to 'anti aging skin care.' It all comes down to being proactive. Skin care that is antiaging slows down the aging process. Here are a few anti-aging skin care suggestions:

1. Adopt good eating habits: Maintaining a proper body metabolism requires a well-balanced diet. Consume a lot of raw fruits and vegetables; they are the best source of fiber and have a highly refreshing effect on the body. Avoid oily and fatty foods; they are deficient in important nutrients and can lead to obesity and other disorders, all of which hasten the aging process.

2. Reduce stress: Probably the most significant anti aging skin care measure is to reduce stress. Stress slows down the aging process by disrupting the body's metabolism. Sleep, exercise, and a relaxing bath are all effective stress relievers. Aromatherapy is also proven to help people relax.

3. Drink plenty of water: It doesn't get any easier than this when it comes to anti aging skin care. Water aids in the removal of toxins from the body, keeping it clean and making it less susceptible to disease. All doctors advocate drinking 8 glasses of water every day.

4. Exercising regularly is an excellent anti-aging skin care treatment. It not only tones your muscles, but it also cleans your skin by emptying out impurities through sweat. To completely remove the toxins, exercise should be followed by a warm shower.

5. When it comes to your skin, stay away from harsh, chemical-based cosmetics. Skin care solutions made from natural ingredients are a wonderful choice. Organic skin care products (either homemade or purchased) can be an extremely effective anti aging skin care solution.

6. Avoid using excessive amounts of skin care products. Both excessive and forceful application is dangerous.

7. Do not neglect skin issues; they might result in lasting harm to the skin. Try over-the-counter medication first, and if it doesn't work, see your dermatologist right away for assistance.

8. Anti-anti aging skin care products containing vitamin C are extremely popular. These, on the other hand, appear to oxidize very quickly (which makes them harmful for the skin). As a result, store them properly. If the product gets a yellowish brown colour, it's because the vitamin C has oxidized and it's no longer safe to use.

9. Protect your skin from UV rays; UV rays have been shown to hasten the aging process. As a result, you should include an excellent sunscreen lotion in your anti aging skin care routine.

CHAPTER SIX

ARE ALL SKIN PROBLEMS SOLVED BY USING NATURAL SKIN CARE PRODUCTS?

When it comes to skin care products, you'll discover that many people are adamant about only utilizing natural products. They see all synthetic goods as skin irritants.

So, are natural skin care products the panacea for all our ills? What if a natural skin care product isn't accessible to treat a certain skin condition? Is it true that synthetic skin care products are so dangerous that they should be prohibited?

People respond to these questions in a variety of ways. However, due to the inclusion of synthetic preservatives, finding a natural skin care product that is 100 percent natural is extremely difficult. Natural skin care products with natural preservatives are available, but their cost may be prohibitive. Furthermore, because such natural skin goods have a shorter shelf life, they are not chosen by natural skin care product makers.

Some people mistakenly believe that because natural skin care products are natural, they cannot hurt the skin. The synthetic or natural nature of a skin care product has no bearing on its suitability. A natural skin care product that isn't right for you can be just as harmful as a synthetic one. So, while you should utilize natural skin care products, you should also be open to synthetic alternatives (you might need them when a natural solution is not available)

Three criteria should be considered while choosing a natural skin care product:

* The skin type of the individual who will use the natural skin care product (dry, oily, normal, sensitive)

* The climate in which it would be utilized, for example, hot and humid conditions would need the usage of oil-free natural skin care products.

* The method for applying and using a natural skin care product. When an excellent natural skin care product (or any product) is not used correctly, it can appear to be ineffective.

You can also make your own natural skin care products using recipes found on the internet and in bookstores.

Organic fruits and vegetables are also often used as a natural skin care treatment. Some essential oils, known as herbal oils, are also beneficial and have moisturizing and antibacterial characteristics.

However, just because you're using a natural skin care product doesn't mean you can ignore other parts of skin care. Natural skin care products should be used as additions to the 'fundamental' suggestions of healthy eating habits (avoiding oily foods), regular exercise, enough of water (8 glasses per day), and hygiene. This will then establish a great and fully natural skin care routine that will assist in the long-term maintenance of healthy, beautiful skin.

CHAPTER SEVEN

CHOOSING A SKIN CARE PRODUCT FOR YOUR FACE

When it comes to skin care, 'facial skin care' appears to be at the top of the list. In the market, there are a plethora of facial skin care products. The most widely utilized facial skin care products are those that are used on a daily basis. Cleansers and moisturizers are examples of these. Toners and exfoliators are also well-known, but few individuals use them for that purpose.

The following criteria are used to classify facial skin care products in general:

* Male or female (so there are facial skin care products for men and there are facial skin care products for women)

* Your skin type (facial skin products for oily skin, facial skin care products for dry skin, facial skin care products for normal skin and facial skin care products for sensitive skin)

* Your age (facial skin care products for old and facial skin care products for young)

* A skin condition (i.e. facial skin care products for treatment of various skin orders like eczema, acne etc)

So that's where you should start looking for a facial skin care product that'll work for you. Identifying your skin type is a fantastic place to start. Also, because skin types change with age, the facial skin product that works for you today may not work for you in the future, therefore you should review the effectiveness of your face skin care product on a regular basis.

Face skin care products come in a variety of forms, such as creams, lotions, gels, masks, and so on, and many individuals try to set one against the other in their debate over which is the best. However, it is impossible to rank one form as superior to another. Really, the greatest face skin care product for you is whatever suits you (and is pleasant for you).

It's crucial to keep in mind, though, that these products function in different ways for different people. So, before using a facial skin care product on a large area of skin, test it on a tiny patch of skin (such as the ear lobes).

Another factor to consider is the condition of your skin. If you have a skin condition of any type, you should seek the opinion of a dermatologist before making a decision and starting to use a facial skin care product.

Once you've chosen a facial skin care product for yourself, you'll need to make sure you use it correctly, which means following proper application practices, using the proper amount, and making the facial product a part of your skin care regimen.

CHAPTER EIGHT

SKIN CARE WITH HERBAL TREATMENT

Skin care is not a new issue; it has been used since ancient times, when herbal skin care was likely the only option to keep skin healthy. Skin care, on the other hand, has undergone a significant transformation. Synthetic/chemical-based skin care procedures have mostly supplanted herbal skin care routines. Herbal skin care recipes, which were formerly ubiquitous, are no longer so popular (and even unknown to a large population). This shift from herbal to synthetic skin care is likely due to two factors: our laziness (or just the quick pace of our life) and the commercialization of skin care. Herbal skin care products have also been made commercially available. Commercial herbal skin care products must be blended with preservatives to extend their shelf life, making them less effective than homemade herbal skin care treatments. However, it appears that things are rapidly changing, with more people choosing for natural and herbal skin care regimens. However, because no one wants to create them at home, the commercial market for herbal skin care products is growing.

So, what exactly are these herbal skin-care mechanisms?

One of the best examples of herbal skin care is Aloe vera, which is an extract from the Aloe plant. Aloe vera, when freshly extracted, is a natural hydrant that aids in skin healing. It also aids in the healing of cuts and the treatment of sunburns.

A variety of herbs have been shown to have cleaning qualities. Such cleansers include dandelion, chamomile, lime blossoms, and rosemary herbs, to name a few. When coupled with other herbs, such as tea, their herbal skin care benefits are activated.

Another significant component of herbal skin care is antiseptics. Herbs that are recognized to have antibacterial effects include lavender, marigold, thyme, and fennel. Rose water and lavender water are also effective toners.

Tea is a key ingredient in herbal skin care. Tea extracts are used to heal skin that has been damaged by ultraviolet light.

Natural skin care oils made from herbal extracts are another option. Some common oils used in herbal skin care are tea tree oil, lavender oil, borage oil, and primrose oil. Fruit oils (for example, extracts from banana, apple, and melon) are used in shower gels (as a hydrating mix)

Homeopathy and aromatherapy are also included in the category of herbal skin care solutions.

Herbal skin care is beneficial not only for nourishing the skin on a daily basis, but also for treating skin illnesses such as eczema and psoriasis. The majority of herbal skin care products have no negative side effects (the most important reason for preferring them over synthetic products) Herbal skin care products are very simple to make at home, making them even more appealing. Herbal skin care is therefore the way to go. This does not, however, imply that you should completely abandon synthetic products. Some folks will argue with their dermatologist if he or she recommends a synthetic product. Accept that some skin conditions may necessitate the use of clinically validated non-herbal skin care products.

CHAPTER NINE

WHICH SHOULD I USE? SKIN CARE CREAMS OR LOTIONS?

The market is brimming with skin-care creams and lotions. Hundreds of skin care creams, lotions, and other items are available for any ailment. The number of skin care products appears to be expanding as a result of continued research and ever-increasing demand. The most common forms in which these treatments are accessible are skin care lotions and skin care creams, and there always seems to be a discussion about which is superior.

To be honest, there is no final solution to this question. It appears to be a matter of personal preference. However, oily creams are unquestionably less popular than non-greasy (or less greasy) creams. Because skin care creams are easier to apply than lotions, they appear to be favoured (over lotions) in situations when the skin care product will not be removed right away. As a result, skin creams appear to be more popular as moisturizers than cleansers or toners. Lotions appear to be favoured over skin care products for toners. Some skin care creams can also be used as toners, but toners are often only available in liquid form. Lotions and skin care creams are both popular for washing; however, lotions appear to be more popular.

Moisturizers are the most popular type of skin care product since they are the most effective at keeping skin moist. Many individuals mistakenly equate skin care lotions with dry and sensitive skin for the same reason. Though this is true to some extent, skin care creams are also used to make products for oily skin, such as vitamin A creams and sulphur creams, which help to reduce the rate of sebum production.

Skin care creams are also used for products that treat skin conditions, particularly those that necessitate the application of a product to a small, localized region. This is owing to the fact that skin care products are easier to administer to the affected region (with less waste). Lotion, on the other hand, is a preferable choice when skin needs to be cleaned with a medicine or substance. Most manufacturers are aware of this, which makes choose between a lotion and a skin care cream easier.

Other skin care creams that are favoured above their lotion counterparts are eye creams and anti-ageing creams.

Knowing how to use your choice (cream or lotion) effectively is more crucial than anything else.

CHAPTER TEN

SKIN CARE FOR MEN

Some guys may be unfamiliar with the term "man skin care." It would have seemed much stranger just a few years ago. However, an increasing number of guys are becoming aware of the significance of man skin care (and hence you see markets flush with man skin care products too). Despite the fact that male and female skins are quite different, 'man skin care' is fairly similar to women's skin care.

Cleaning is the first step in 'man skin care.' Cleansers that dissolve in water are advised. Cleaning the skin removes dirt, grease, and pollutants, as well as preventing pore clogging. Because of the oily nature of male skin, cleaning is an important aspect of the man skin care routine. Cleaning should be done at least once a day, and twice a day is much better. It's not a good idea to use soap on your face.

Shaving is a big part of 'man skin care.' One of the most significant guy skin care items is shaving foam/gel/cream and after shave lotion. A suitable selection of shaving-related equipment and products is required for serious 'man skin care.' The skin type should be one of the most important factors to consider when selecting shaving products (since the degree of oiliness differs from person to person). Aftershaves containing alcohol should be avoided. Man skin care also necessitates the usage of high-quality razors. Swivel-head razors are recommended in this situation since they are known to reduce cuts. Aside from these products and equipment, you must also use them correctly. When using your razor, be gentle. Avoid scratching your skin; instead, employ a gentle, smooth motion (after all, it's about eliminating hair, not the skin).

Due to bigger pores and more active sebaceous glands, male skin is thicker and oilier than female skin. Regular shaving, on the other hand, can easily dry the skin. As a result, moisturisers are an important aspect of men's skin care. After shaving, a moisturizing gel or lotion should be applied. Some shaving foams/gels, in fact, have a built-in moisturizing function. Moisturizers should be lightly patted over the face and massaged gently upwards.

Using a sunscreen is a vital male skin care measure, even though a guy's skin is less susceptible to skin cancer caused by UV radiation. Use a moisturiser that has both a sunscreen and a moisturising effect.

Another fantastic alternative for 'man skin care' is to utilize products that have natural ingredients such as aloe vera, sea salt, and coconut, among others. Natural antibacterial oils, such as lavender and tea tree, are also beneficial for men's skin care.

Skin care for men is not as difficult as many men believe. It requires only a few minutes of your time each day in order to provide you with healthy skin in the present and future.

CHAPTER ELEVEN

SKIN CARE THAT IS ORGANIC

"If something can be done naturally, why use artificial means?" is the underlying principle of "organic skin care." The most natural form of 'skin care' is organic skin care. In fact, when man first became aware of his skin's needs, 'organic skin care' was likely the first product he used. Organic skin care is not only better for your skin, but it is also less expensive. Organic skin care, when practiced correctly, can help avoid the formation of many skin illnesses and keep your skin healthy and youthful-looking for a much longer period of time.

Organic fruits and vegetables are the most commonly used ingredients in organic skin care routines; for example, cucumber is frequently used in organic skin care routines. Turmeric, apple, papaya, and ginger are just a few examples of organic skin care ingredients. These natural materials provide a revitalizing and rejuvenating impact on your skin. Organic skin care is included in almost every skin care book or reference (including the actions of various fruits and vegetables on skin). So pick the ones that are better suited to your skin type and begin experimenting with them until you find the ones that are best suited for your organic skin care routine. It's critical to use organic fruits and vegetables that are fresh. Don't try to use the rotten ones for your skin; the garbage bin is their only home.

Milk is known for its cleansing effects; in fact, the word 'milk' appears in the names of various skin care products. A mixture of milk and ground oats work wonders as a cleanser.

Ground oatmeal is a common element in organic skin care regimens since it is especially helpful for oily skin. It's used to make organic facial packs in various combinations, such as with egg, honey, milk, and fruits.

Another element in organic skin care techniques is wheat germ. It's high in vitamin E and known for its exfoliating and moisturizing effects. Wheat germ is used to make face masks for normal and dry skin types in various combinations with other organic components. Wheat germ oil is another organic skin care product made from wheat germ.

Other organic compounds that are famous for their exfoliating and moisturizing characteristics include yogurt and sour cream.

Organic honey is frequently used in organic skin care methods. It aids in the preservation of moisture and gives skin a healthy glow.

In organic skin care treatments, rose water is used as a toner. Lavender water is also very popular.

The term "organic skin care" refers to the use of a variety of organic elements that complement and increase each other's effectiveness. Furthermore, these combinations aid in overcoming the negative effects (if any) of the numerous organic elements that make them up.

Organic skin care is a true art form that, once mastered, can produce amazing results at a low cost.

CHAPTER TWELVE

'PERSONAL SKIN CARE' IS A SET OF PROCEDURES THAT MUST BE FOLLOWED RELIGIOUSLY

We're all aware of the significance of 'personal skin care.' Individual perspectives on how-to (for personal skin care) differ. Some people consider visiting to a beauty salon every other day to be personal skin care. Others feel that personal skin care is simply a question of periodically putting a cream or lotion to your skin. Then there are many who believe that personal skin care is a once-a-month or once-a-year event. Others are constantly preoccupied with 'personal skin care.' Personal skin care, on the other hand, is neither difficult nor expensive (considering how beneficial it is). Personal skin care entails adhering to a schedule or procedure for responding to your skin's needs.

Before you begin a program, you must first assess your skin type (oily, dry, sensitive, normal, etc.) and choose personal skin care products that are appropriate for it (you might have to experiment with a few personal skin care products). This is a practice that most people with regular skin should be able to follow.

'Cleansing' is the first step in any personal skin care routine. Oil, water, and surfactants are the three main elements of a cleaner (wetting agents). Dirt and oil are extracted from your skin by oil and surfactants, which are then flushed out by water, leaving your skin clean. It's possible that you'll have to try a few different cleansers before you find the one that works best for you. You should, however, always use soap-free cleansers. You should also clean with Luke warm water (hot and cold water, both, cause damage to your skin). Make sure you don't over-cleanse your skin and wind up harming it.

Exfoliation is the second step in a personal skin care routine. The skin has a natural maintenance mechanism that involves removing dead cells and replacing them with new ones. Exfoliation is simply a method of assisting the skin in this process. Although dead skin cells are unable to respond to personal skin care products, they nevertheless devour them, preventing the products from reaching new skin cells. As a result, eliminating dead skin cells is critical to improving the efficacy of all personal skin care products. Exfoliation is usually done immediately after cleansing. It's critical to understand how much exfoliation you require, like with any particular skin care technique. For oily/normal skin, exfoliate 4-5 times per week; for dry/sensitive skin, exfoliate 1-2 times per week. In hot and humid temperatures, exfoliate a couple of times more.

Moisturizers are the next step in your personal skin care program. One of the most crucial aspects of personal skin care is this. Moisturizers are necessary even for those with oily skin. Moisturizers not only seal moisture in your skin cells, but they also draw moisture from the air when it's needed. Overuse of moisturizer, on the other hand, can block skin pores and injure your skin. Within one week of using the moisturiser, the amount of moisturiser required by your skin will become obvious. It's also ideal to apply the moisturizer while your skin is still damp.

Sunscreen is the last step in your personal skin care routine. Many moisturizers (day-time creams/moisturizers) include UV protection, allowing you to reap double benefits. These types of moisturizers should be used on a daily basis (irrespective of whether it is sunny or cloudy).

Experiment with different personal skin care products as well as the amount of product you need to apply. The greatest personal skin care recipe for you is what provides you the best results. If you have a skin problem, however, you should see a dermatologist before utilizing any personal skin care products.

CHAPTER THIRTEEN

SKIN CARE THAT IS SERIOUS BUSINESS

'Serious skin care' is all about keeping your skin healthy and radiant for the rest of your life. Your body's natural skin-care processes deteriorate as you age. So, 'serious skin care' is about adapting to your skin's changing needs. As a result, 'serious skin care' entails evaluating, analyzing, and altering your skin care practices on a regular basis. The environment, your age, and changes in your skin type should all influence your skin care program.

'Serious skin care' also entails a level of attentiveness. Every day, more and more truths are revealed because to technical developments and research. In addition, the makeup and nature of skin care products appear to be evolving with time. As a result, trying out new products is an important aspect of serious skin care. However, 'serious skin care' recommends testing a new product on a small patch of skin (not your face) initially to see how it reacts.

Knowing how to utilize your skin care products is also part of 'serious skin care.' Applying moisturizers when the skin is damp, using upward strokes for greater penetration of skin care products, removing make-up before night, washing before moisturising or applying make-up, using the appropriate amount of skin care products, and so on are all good practices. As a result, another major area of serious skin care is enhancing the effectiveness of your skin care products.

Serious skin care also includes some precautions, such as avoiding contact with detergents. Serious skin care entails treating your skin with attention. Over-exfoliation, the use of low-quality products, and the usage of strong-chemical-based treatments are all bad for your skin.

Some people have a misunderstanding regarding the importance of serious skin care. Serious skin care for them entails using big quantities of products as frequently as feasible. However, this isn't serious skin care (thus the importance of raising awareness).

Visiting your dermatologist for treatment of skin issues is also part of 'serious skin care.' Ignoring skin problems can be harmful to your skin and result in lasting damage. If things don't improve with over-the-counter medication, you should see a dermatologist right away. Self-surgery, such as squeezing acne or pimples, is a no-no (it can lead to permanent damage of your skin).

So, when it comes to serious skin care, it's all about protection and prevention (than treatment). It's important to be proactive as well as reactive when it comes to skin care. In fact, we may argue that 'serious skin care' is about being proactive about your skin's needs so that you don't have to be reactive as much.

CHAPTER FOURTEEN

COSMETICS FOR SKIN CARE: ARE THEY BENEFICIAL OR HARMFUL?

A glowing, healthy complexion boosts one's self-esteem. Some people are inherently attractive and hence do not require the use of any 'skin care cosmetics.' Others, on the other hand, do not apply skin care cosmetics because they are lazy. Some people believe that skin care cosmetics can hurt their skin and hence avoid using any type of skin care cosmetic. However, a big number of people utilize skin care cosmetics (which is why the skin care cosmetics industry is thriving).

Is skin care cosmetic beneficial or harmful? Well, it appears that there are differing viewpoints. One thing is certain, however: looking gorgeous is unquestionably appealing. Furthermore, using too much skin care cosmetic can be dangerous (as such, excess of anything is harmful). So, what's a person to do?

The first step is to create (and stick to) a skin care program that will keep your skin looking healthy and disease-free. Cleanse and moisturize every day, and tone and exfoliate once in a while, is the typical guideline (as and when needed).

Then there's the skin care product that you'll be using as well (as beauty enhancers). These skin care products can be used as part of your daily regimen or solely on special occasions (e.g. when attending a party etc).

The most crucial aspect of skin care cosmetics is their choosing. Here are some guidelines to follow while choosing a skin care product:

* As a general rule, use cosmetics that are appropriate for your skin type. This is true for both everyday items and skin care cosmetics. So, look at the label to see what it says, such as 'for dry skin exclusively' or 'for all skin types,' and so on.

* Before using a skin care product, give it a test run. This can be accomplished by applying the skin care cosmetic to a small piece of skin, such as the earlobes, and observing how your skin reacts to it.

* Look for substances that you are allergic to in the skin care cosmetic's ingredients. Use skin-harming items sparingly, such as cosmetics with high alcohol concentrations; such cosmetics may work temporarily but cause long-term damage to your skin.

* 'More isn't always better.' Make sure you use the proper amount of products (neither less not more). Also, be gentle with your skin and apply skin care products according to the manufacturer's instructions. Rubbing too hard or attempting to squeeze a pimple might cause irreversible skin damage.

* Finally, if you have a skin condition such as acne, you should get advice from a doctor before using any skin care product.

CHAPTER FIFTEEN

THE SIGNIFICANCE OF TAKING CARE OF YOUR SKIN

"Packaging is as crucial as the gift itself," as most gift manufacturing firms will tell you. The same can be said for you. Your skin, or outer-self, is just as significant as your inner-self. Many people are aware of the importance of skin care. This is one of the reasons why there are so many skin care products on the market, and most of them seem to work very well. We tend to link skin care with just looking beautiful. But there's a lot more to it than that. There are numerous advantages to having healthy, bright skin.

To begin with, it has a positive impact on you. It helps you feel revitalized and energized. You are able to do more tasks and are more efficient in all you do. More significantly, the freshness enhances your pleasure and brightens your day. As a result, having healthy skin contributes to self-assurance. Yes, you may take the most of the credit for doing it (however, do leave a little for the skin care products too).

Furthermore, the flow of pleasant energy is felt by those around you, and you notice that they are also friendlier with you. Others will respect you more. They respond to your questions more quickly. They can sense the freshness that you exude. They enjoy collaborating with and for you. That is, in fact, how it works. Some people may even inquire about the skin care products you employ (you might or might not reveal those secret skin care products to them). As a result, having good skin can help you create a pleasant and friendly workplace. Carelessness or negligence on this front, on the other hand, might make you appear unappealing and dull. Not only will you appear dull, but you will also feel dull. Your productivity has suffered as a result of this. It's possible that the folks you meet will not be as friendly. In fact, it could cause the aging process to begin considerably earlier.

As a result, the significance of skin care cannot be overstated. Skin care, on the other hand, is not difficult at all. There are numerous skin care products to pick from, and you can select the ones that best fit your needs. Skin care products are categorised in a variety of ways, and understanding these classifications can help you better understand them and make a decision.

* The first classification is based on skin type; for example, there are skin care products for oily skin, skin care products for dry skin, skin care products for sensitive skin, and so forth.

* Another option is to categorize skin care products based on their intended function, such as moisturisers, cleansers, exfoliating products, toners, and so on.

* Then there are skin care products for acne, stretch marks, anti-aging, and other skin problems.

* Another classification is based on the ingredients, such as herbal skin care, synthetic skin care, cosmetic skin care, and so on.

Skin care products, on the other hand, are not the only approach to care for your skin. You should also incorporate some basic skin-care procedures into your daily routine.

CHAPTER SIXTEEN

THE MOST COMMON SKIN CONDITIONS TREATED WITH SKIN CARE PRODUCTS.

A glowing and healthy skin is an asset. Skin is not only about appearance, but also about health. As a result, skin care treatment should be taken seriously. If you have a skin problem, you should seek out the suitable skin care treatment. For any skin problem, skin care treatment begins with steps targeted at preventing the disorder (what we can also call as proactive or preventive skin care treatment). Preventive/proactive skin care treatment consists of developing and following fundamental skin care regimens. Even if you've followed this preventive skin care regimen, skin diseases can still arise. Preventive skin care simply minimizes the likelihood of recurrence. Let's look at some of the most prevalent skin problems and how they're treated.

One of the most prevalent issues is acne. The first form of skin care treatment, once again, is to control acne and prevent it from worsening. As a result, avoid wearing tight clothing, which is known to induce body acne by trapping sweat. If you keep touching the imperfections (rather don't even touch them at all), you may end up exacerbating the condition. Also, avoid scrubbing or squeezing them too hard. Mild cleansers are a recommended acne skin care treatment. Acne can be treated more quickly using an over-the-counter skin care solution.

The treatment of dry skin is usually simple. Moisturizers, when used correctly and in the appropriate amounts, are the most effective skin care treatment for dry skin. Apply moisturiser when your skin is still damp for optimal effects. Applying too much or too little moisturizer is also a no-no. If you don't see any improvements after 3-4 weeks, you may need to see your dermatologist for dry skin therapy.

Overexposure to UV radiation causes brown patches on sun-exposed parts of skin, such as the face and hands. Use a sunscreen lotion with a high SPF (sun protection factor), such as 15, as a skin care therapy for brown spots. Regardless of the weather (sunny or gloomy), this should be used. Covering up exposed parts with clothing (caps, full-sleeved shirts/t-shirts, and umbrella) is another sort of skin care treatment.

Also, if your basic skin care treatment or over-the-counter medication isn't working, you should see a dermatologist for expert skin care therapy right away. You should also tell the doctor about any skin care treatments you've had up to that point. So bring the most up-to-date information about skin care treatments (and products) with you. The dermatologist will prescribe a skin care therapy based on your skin condition and the details of your previous skin care treatment, such as oral antibiotics, chemical peels, and retinoid, and you will be on your path to recovery.

CHAPTER SEVENTEEN

THE TRUTH ABOUT CARING FOR OILY SKIN

To begin discussing oily skin care, it's critical to first comprehend the causes of oily skin. Simply said, oily skin is the result of excessive sebum production (an oily substance that is naturally produced by skin). Excess of anything is bad, as we all know, and excessive sebum is no exception. It causes skin pores to clog, resulting in the accumulation of dead cells and, as a result, the production of pimples/acne. Furthermore, greasy skin degrades your appearance. As a result, 'oily skin care' is just as necessary as 'skin care' for other skin types.

The primary goal of "oily skin care" is to get rid of excess sebum or oil on the skin. Oily skin care techniques, on the other hand, should not result in full oil elimination. The use of a cleanser is the first step in 'oily skin care.' However, not all cleansers are effective. You'll need a cleanser that contains salicylic acid, a beta-hydroxy acid that slows down the production of sebum. It is recommended that you cleanse twice a day (and even more in hot and humid conditions).

The majority of oily skin care products are oil-free; however, it is always a good idea to examine the product's contents before purchasing it. This is especially true if the product is labelled as "appropriate for all skin types" rather than "oily skin care product." If you aren't overly oily, several of these 'suitable for all' products may work for you as well. Only oily skin care products are acceptable for severely oily skin. An alcohol-based toner can be used in your oily skin care routine (for an extremely oily skin). After cleansing, this can be the second step in your oily skin care program. Excessive toning, on the other hand, can be harmful to your skin.

A light moisturiser can be used as the following step in your oily skin care routine. If you need to include this in your oily skin care routine, it will depend on the degree of oiliness of your skin. If you do decide to apply a moisturizer, make sure it's oil-free, wax-free, and lipid-free.

As an oily skin care measure, you might use a clay mask once a week.

When it comes to oily skin care products, you may need to try a few before finding one that is truly perfect for your skin.

If these measures do not yield the desired results, get guidance from a qualified dermatologist. He could prescribe harsher oily skin care treatments, such as vitamin A creams, retinoids, sulphur creams, and so on, to help with oily skin problems.

CHAPTER EIGHTEEN

THE DRY SKIN CARE RECIPE

Dry skin is a problem that must be addressed. Dry skin causes the upper layer of skin to crack, giving it an unpleasant appearance. Dry skin is caused by a dry atmosphere, hormonal changes, excessive exfoliation, and the treatment of other skin conditions. Furthermore, dryness may be a natural characteristic of one's skin. Whatever the reason, 'dry skin care' is critical (but not very difficult).

Moisturizers, the most effective cure for dry skin, are the first step in 'dry skin care.' Moisturizers are often divided into two groups based on how they provide 'dry skin care.'

The first group comprises moisturisers such as Vaseline, which provide 'dry skin care' simply by retaining moisture within the skin. These moisturizers are reasonably priced and widely available (even at grocery shops).

Moisturizers that extract moisture from the environment and provide it to the skin fall into the second type. In humid environments, this is a particularly efficient method of 'dry skin care.' Humectants are the moisturisers that give this type of 'dry skin care.' As much as possible, you should use a non-greasy moisturiser for effective dry skin care. Humectants are a type of non greasy moisturizer. Humectants include propylene glycol, urea, glycerine, and hyaluronic acid, among others.

'Dry skin care' entails not only the application of moisturizers, but also the appropriate application of such moisturizers. Cleansing the skin before applying moisturizer is the finest 'dry skin care technique.' Apply the moisturiser while the skin is still damp to make your 'dry skin care' even more effective (after cleansing). Also, make sure you're using non-soap items (especially on your face, neck and arms). Exfoliation aids in the care of dry skin by eliminating dead skin cells. However, don't scrub your skin too aggressively. Sun protection should be a part of your dry skin care treatments and products. Avoid excessive and direct sun exposure (by using an umbrella/hat, for example). Before going out, use a decent sunscreen lotion. Many moisturizers also give UV protection as well as dry skin care.

You can also get natural 'dry skin care' products, which are items that provide 'dry skin care' in a natural method (without the use of synthetic chemicals). These dry skin care solutions provide lipid improvements to the skin, allowing the skin to retain moisture. Another crucial aspect of 'dry skin care' is the water temperature you use in the shower or when washing your face – use warm water; too hot or cold water can also create dryness.

'Dry skin care' also entails treating your skin with care. Harsh detergents and alcohol-based cleaners should be avoided. Also, do not wipe your face with your towel after a face wash; instead, gently pat it to absorb the water.

Dry skin care is, on the whole, very straightforward for anyone who takes it seriously.

CHAPTER NINETEEN

MAKE-UP AND SKIN-CARE ADVICE

Make-up and skin care are typically seen to be a woman's forte. Men rarely bother with 'make-up and skin care.' Many guys take care of their skin, but make-up is a foreign concept to them. It wouldn't make sense to treat make-up and skin care as separate topics; after all, make-up will only function if the skin is healthy. So, how do you combine make-up and skin care in your routine? Here are some make-up and skin-care suggestions:

* Always keep skin care in mind while purchasing cosmetics or applying them to your skin after purchase. So you're buying a 'make-up and skin-care' product rather than just a make-up item. Examine the ingredients to see if there are any items that you may be allergic to. Check to see whether it includes chemicals in high concentrations that could hurt your skin.

* 'Make-up and skin care' also entails putting products to the test before utilizing them. Apply the makeup to a small section of skin, such as your earlobes, and see how your skin reacts.

* Keep track of the expiration dates on your cosmetics and never use them after they have passed their expiration date. In reality, some items (such as vitamin C-based products) spoil far sooner than their expiration dates if they are not properly stored.

* Cleanliness is crucial in the application of make-up and skin care products. Regularly sharpen your eyeliners, and keep all of your cosmetic tools clean at all times. You may schedule an overhaul of your

equipment once a month. Cleanliness should also entail keeping your hair clean at all times as part of your make-up and skin-care routine.

* Another vital part of make-up and skin care is nail care. Use high-quality nail polish and keep your nails clean at all times. After you've finished washing and polishing your nails, apply cuticle oil to the edges of your nails.

* Instead of using a pencil eye liner, use a liquid eye liner if you have deep-set eyes. This will prevent smearing at your eyelid's deep edges.

* If you have a skin condition, such as acne, avoid wearing heavy or chemical-based make-up. If you're unsure about which make-up products you can use while dealing with acne or another skin condition, go to your dermatologist. Squeezing pimples/acne is never a good idea. Keep in mind that make-up and skin care should not be incompatible.

* Remove your make-up with a gentle cleanser (instead of just washing it away).

* The golden rule of "never sleep with your make-up on" is another crucial "make-up and skin care" method.

* When applying deodorant, keep the required distance between the nozzle and your skin in mind (as mentioned on the deodorant pack).

As a result, make-up and skin care should constantly be combined. Makeup and skin care should not be treated separately.

CHAPTER TWENTY

TOP TEN SKIN-CARE SUGGESTIONS

One of the most crucial factors for beauty improvement is healthy skin. This post on skin care tips is an attempt to provide you with the top ten skin care suggestions. The number of skin care suggestions has been limited to ten since any more would be difficult to remember and would obscure the more significant skin care tips. So, here are the top 10 skin care suggestions:

* One of the most crucial skin care tips is to know your skin type. This is critical because not all skin care products are suitable for everyone. In truth, all skin care products state which skin types they are intended for.

'Drink a lot of water,' says the adage. This will not only keep your skin moisturized, but it will also aid in the overall health of your body (and in turn your skin). This may appear strange to some, but it is a vital skin care advice.

* Cleanse your skin on a regular basis (1-2 times every day). This is a really powerful skin care method for removing dirt and other harsh materials from your skin. Cleaning is especially crucial after being away from home for an extended period of time (and hence exposed to pollutants, dust etc). This skin care advice also recommends cleaning with Luke warm water (hot and cold water, both, cause damage to your skin)

* Be gentle with yourself; after all, it's your skin. Scrub/exfoliate gently and infrequently. Applying too much or too many skin care products is also a bad idea. This is a must-follow skin-care tip.

* Always keep your skin moisturized. This is one of the most crucial skin-care suggestions. Do not allow your skin to become dry. The surface layer of your skin breaks down as a result of dryness, giving you a harsh and unpleasant appearance. Use emollients/moisturizers. Moisturizers are most effective when applied on wet skin.

* Avoid washing your face with soap. Soap should be used just from the neck down. This is a simple but vital piece of skin-care advice.

* Protect yourself from the sun's harmful UV rays by wearing sunscreen. You can use sunscreen-infused daytime moisturizers to your skin. Even if it's cloudy, use them. Because UV rays are known to cause skin cancer, this skin care tip should be followed religiously.

* Not only for skin care, but for overall health, a little exercise and a good night's sleep are also vital. Sleep deprivation can develop wrinkles beneath the eyes, and a lack of activity can cause your skin to sag. Exercise and sleep are also beneficial in reducing stress. So, in addition to being a skin care tip, this is a health care tip as well.

* Handle skin problems with caution. This skin-care tip emphasizes the importance of not neglecting any skin problems. Before you start using a skin care product, talk to your dermatologist (lest you do end up harming your skin even more).

* Get rid of stress. Although everyone is aware of the negative effects of stress, it is sometimes necessary to state the obvious (and hence this skin care tip found its place here). Yes, stress has a negative impact on the skin. So, take a break, relax in a warm bubble bath, or simply get some rest.

CHAPTER TWENTY ONE

THE CHALLENGE OF VITAMIN C SKIN CARE

Vitamin C is frequently recognized as an anti-aging or wrinkle-fighting substance. In technical words, the fundamental goal of 'Vitamin C skin care' is to enhance collagen synthesis (a structural protein that is found in skin). The ability of 'Vitamin C skin care' to counteract free radicals, which cause skin damage, is an additional benefit.

Vitamin C skin care, on the other hand, is currently facing a significant problem. This is due to Vitamin C skin care products' proclivity for oxidation. The Vitamin C in Vitamin C skin care products is oxidized when it comes into touch with any oxidizing factor (e.g. air), rendering the Vitamin C skin care product worthless (in fact counter-effective). The oxidized Vitamin C gives the Vitamin C skin care product a yellowish-brown color. Before purchasing a Vitamin C skin care product, make sure to check this. Even after you've purchased a Vitamin C skin care product, be sure it's stored properly and that it's still usable (i.e. it hasn't turned yellowish-brown).

Manufacturers of Vitamin C skin care products have attempted to address this (oxidation) issue in a variety of methods (and research on Vitamin C skin care products is on the top of their list). Maintaining a high concentration (say 10%) of Vitamin C in skin care products is one way to sustain their effectiveness for a long time. However, this raises the price of Vitamin C skin care products. Vitamin C skin care products are already reasonably priced, and increasing their price will put product producers out of business. The usage of Vitamin C derivatives is another option (like ascorbyl palmitate and magnesium ascorbyl phosphate). Not only are they more sturdy, but they're also less expensive. Even though derivatives-based skin care products aren't as effective as Vitamin C skin care products, their oxidation resistance is a desirable feature that makes them appealing. Furthermore, these are said to be less annoying.

When it comes to the efficacy of Vitamin C skin care products, it's vital to remember that not everyone responds to the treatment. So it's not a magical elixir at all. If you don't see any changes in your skin, it's possible that your skin isn't responding to the Vitamin C therapy (and the Vitamin C skin care products might not be at fault, at all).

As additional study is done, we can only cross our fingers and wait for a complete solution to the problems that 'Vitamin C skin care' is currently facing.

CHAPTER TWENTY TWO

WHAT IS NATURAL SKIN CARE?

Simply put, 'natural skin care' is the process of caring for your skin without the use of chemicals. Natural skin care encourages allowing the skin to look after itself (without the use of synthetic products or chemicals). 'Natural skin care' refers to the development of beneficial habits in your daily routine. Many natural skin care methods are similar to those used for body care in general.

Let's have a look at what these natural skin care methods are.

'Drink a lot of water,' is the first and most important natural skin care measure. Every day, you should drink at least 8 glasses of water. Water assists in the natural removal of toxins from the body. It aids in the body's overall maintenance and improves the health of all organs (not just skin).

Another low-cost method of natural skin care is general cleaning. General cleanliness includes taking a daily shower, wearing clean clothes, and sleeping on a clean mattress/pillow. After all, keeping your skin clean is the key to avoiding skin problems.

The next step is to start exercising regularly. Exercise promotes blood flow, which aids in the removal of toxins from the body and keeps you healthy. Exercise can also aid in the reduction of stress, which is the number one enemy of good health.

Natural skin care also includes consuming healthy foods and adopting good eating habits. Some foods (for example, oily foods) are known to cause acne and should be avoided whenever feasible. Your diet should be a well-balanced combination of nutrient-dense foods. Raw fruits and vegetables are believed to provide your body a boost of energy and aid in the elimination of pollutants.

A good night's sleep is also essential for good health and overcoming stress. A good night's sleep prevents skin from slackening as a natural skin care measure.

Another natural skin care therapy is to reduce stress. Stress has a negative impact on the body and health. Drinking enough of water, getting enough sleep, and exercising have all been recommended as stress relievers. Stress can also be relieved by taking a warm bath, listening to music, or participating in your favorite sport. Yoga is yet another stress-relieving technique that is rapidly gaining popularity among the general public.

Another natural skin care method is to avoid excessive sun exposure (by wearing long-sleeved clothing, a helmet, and an umbrella, for example). Sunscreen creams are also advised if needed.

Many traditional and home-made natural skin care products/measures are also well-known for their efficacy. Such steps are not only natural and simple to implement, but they are also reasonably priced.

Aside from that, the commercial sector has a plethora of natural skin care products. These include things like lavender oil, aloe vera, and other natural remedies that have no negative side effects.

CHAPTER TWENTY THREE

CHOOSING THE BEST SKIN CARE PRODUCT

There's nothing quite like the best skin care product. There can't possibly be such a thing as "the best skin care product," because everyone's skin care needs are different (based on the skin type to some extent). For example, a product that is the "greatest skin care product" for one individual may be the worst for another. 'What is the best skin care product for my skin type?' is a more logical question to ask. However, this isn't entirely reasonable. People are usually divided into four categories based on their skin types: dry skin, oily skin, normal skin, and sensitive skin. This classification, however, is far too wide to be utilized to determine the best skin care product. We can say things like "best skin care product for dry skin" or "best skin care product for oily skin" instead of just "best skin care product." But that is exactly what it is - 'better'; it is still inaccurate.

As a result, the question should be rephrased as 'What is the best skin care product for me?' Yes, this is the precise question you should be asking, and unfortunately, there is no simple solution. It will take some work on your part to find the ideal skin care product for yourself.

First and foremost, you must comprehend how skin care products function. This is straightforward. All skin care products can be divided into two categories: active and inert components. The active substances are those that have a direct effect on your skin. The inactive substances just aid in the delivery of the active elements to your skin. In order for the product to be effective, both of the ingredients must be beneficial to your skin (and move on to become the best skin care product for you).

The manner you apply your skin care products is just as crucial as the ingredients. This is, in fact, considerably more critical. If you don't know how to use skin care products properly, you may spend your entire life looking for the ideal skin care product for yourself, even if it has already passed you by. Furthermore, deciding on the frequency of application is crucial (of the skin care product). The selection of the best skin care product is also influenced by environmental conditions such as temperature, humidity, and pollution levels. Here are some guidelines to follow to make sure your best skin care product is truly the best for you:

* Before you apply the best skin care product, make sure your skin is clean.

* Remove your makeup with a makeup remover rather than plain water before going to bed.

* When active components are put over another product, such as a moisturizer, their effectiveness is diminished. So start with your best skin care product and then add some moisturizer if needed.

* Use the items on skin that is moist and heated.

* You'll have to try a few different products before deciding the best skin care product for you.

* Don't scrub too hard or too much.

* Change your skin care routine according to the seasons (winter/summer, etc.), environmental variables, and your skin type.

It's important to remember that finding the perfect skin care product doesn't happen quickly. The only way to find the 'Best skin care product' is to try (and be attentive to you).

9 798419 873803